CANNABIS COOKBOOK

MAIN COURSE – 80+ Quick and easy to prepare at home recipes, step-by-step guide to the best cannabis recipes- THC infused recipes

TABLE OF CONTENTS

BREAKFAST	7
FRENCH TOAST	7
HUEVOS TOSTADAS	8
SANDWICHES	10
GRILLED CHEESE SANDWICH	11
HAM & CHEDDAR PANINI	12
WAFFLES	13
BISCUITS	14
CRISPY BACON	16
MUNCHIE BALLS	17
QUESADILLA	18
FOIE GRAS PATE	19
STEAK WITH CHIMICHURRI SAUCE	20
MUSHROOM BRUSCHETTA	21
GNOCCHI IN GANJA BUTTER	22
CHICKEN PASTA	24
LOBSTER ETOUFFEE	25
SHRIMP SCAMPI	27
STRIP STEAK	28
HOT WINGS	29
MAC AND CHEESE	30
TACOS	31
BURGERS	32
SALAD	33
TURKEY BOLOGNESE	35

BATTERED FISH	36
TUNA POKE BOWL	38
STEAK SALAD	40
BAKED BEANS	41
STUFFED POTATOES	42
SHRIMP QUESADILLA	44
LUNCH	46
SPINACH, ARTICHOKE & MUSHROOM FETTUCCINE	46
QUINOA KALE SALAD	47
LEMON CHICKEN	49
SWEET CORN SALAD	50
ROASTED MUSHROOMS	51
HOT WINGS	53
BACON AND CHEESE POTATOES	54
BROCCOLI QUICHE	55
SPINACH QUICHE	56
BUTTERNUT SQUASH SOUP	58
PUMPKIN POTATO SOUP	59
TOMATO SOUP	61
QUINOA STEW	62
CHILI CON	64
PEA SOUP	65
FRENCH ONION SOUP	67
SPICY BURGERS	68
VEGGIE TART	70
AVOCADO SHRIMP SALAD	71

GAZPACHO	72
SNACKS, DRINKS & DIPS	74
MUDDY BUDDIES	74
CARAMELS	75
FUDGE	76
BROWNIES	77
COOKIE BARS	78
BROWNIE BARS	79
INDIAN BHANG	80
AVOCADO SHAKE	81
BLUEBERRIES SMOOTHIE	82
HOT CHOCOLATE	83
ICED TEA	84
CARROT, BEET JUICE	85
BLOODY MARY	86
COCONANABERRY SMOOTHIE	87
MARTINI	88
VANILLA MILKSHAKE	89
APPLE CIDER	90
PEAR PROSECCO	91
CANNABIS SYRUP	92
PEANUT BUTTER MILKSHAKE	93
NUT BUTTER	94
STRAWBERRY JAM	95
VINAIGRETTE	96
SALAD DRESSING	97

GUACAMOLE	98
CUCUMBER DIP	99
CANNAQUESO DIP	100
HUMMUS	101
SPINACH DIP	102
BLUE CHEESE DIP	103

Copyright 2018 by Noah Jerris - All rights reserved.

This document is geared towards providing exact and reliable information in regards to the topic and issue covered. The publication is sold with the idea that the publisher is not required to render accounting, officially permitted, or otherwise, qualified services. If advice is necessary, legal or professional, a practiced individual in the profession should be ordered.

- From a Declaration of Principles which was accepted and approved equally by a Committee of the American Bar Association and a Committee of Publishers and Associations.

In no way is it legal to reproduce, duplicate, or transmit any part of this document in either electronic means or in printed format. Recording of this publication is strictly prohibited and any storage of this document is not allowed unless with written permission from the publisher. All rights reserved.

The information provided herein is stated to be truthful and consistent, in that any liability, in terms of inattention or otherwise, by any usage or abuse of any policies, processes, or directions contained within is the solitary and utter responsibility of the recipient reader. Under no circumstances will any legal responsibility or blame be held against the publisher for any reparation, damages, or monetary loss due to the information herein, either directly or indirectly.

Respective authors own all copyrights not held by the publisher.

The information herein is offered for informational purposes solely, and is universal as so. The presentation of the information is without contract or any type of guarantee assurance.

The trademarks that are used are without any consent, and the publication of the trademark is without permission or backing by the trademark owner. All trademarks and brands within this book are for clarifying purposes only and are the owned by the owners themselves, not affiliated with this document.

Introduction

Cannabis recipes for personal enjoyment but also for family enjoyment. You will love them for sure for how easy it is to prepare them.

BREAKFAST

FRENCH TOAST

Serves: **4**

Prep Time: **8** Hours

Cook Time: **50** Minutes

Total Time: **8h 50** Minutes

INGREDIENTS

- ¼ cup sugar
- 4 tbs cannabis-infused butter
- 4 eggs
- 3 tbs maple syrup
- 1 ½ tsp vanilla
- 1 french baguette
- 2 tbs butter
- 1 tsp salt
- 1 cup milk

DIRECTIONS

1. **Butter a baking dish.**

2. Slice the baguette.
3. Mix the butters until combined.
4. Spread the butter onto a side of each slice.
5. Place the slices on the baking dish.
6. Whisk the eggs, milk, vanilla, salt, syrup, and sugar in a bowl.
7. Pour the mixture over the bread slices.
8. Refrigerate for 8 hours.
9. Bake for 50 minutes at 350F.
10. Serve dusted with powdered sugar.

HUEVOS TOSTADAS

Serves: 2
Prep Time: 10 Minutes
Cook Time: 15 Minutes
Total Time: 25 Minutes

INGREDIENTS

- 3 tbs cannabis-infused oil
- 1 onion
- Thyme

- 1 ½ cup cooked rice
- 4 tostada shells
- 2 eggs
- 3 tbs cheese
- Hot sauce
- ½ cup cilantro
- 1 ½ tbs cannabis-infused oil
- 1 ½ tsp chili powder
- 1 tsp cumin
- Salt
- 1 cup cabbage
- ½ cup celery
- Pepper

DIRECTIONS

1. Heat 2 tbs of cannabis oil.
2. Saute the onions for 10 minutes.
3. Add the celery, cabbage and thyme and saute for another 5 minutes.
4. Mix the rice, chili, 1 tbs oil, cilantro, cumin, salt and pepper.
5. Divide the rice on top of each tostada.
6. Place the cabbage on top.
7. Fry the eggs.
8. Place the fried eggs on top.
9. Serve with hot sauce.

SANDWICHES

Serves: **4**

Prep Time: **5** Minutes

Cook Time: **5** Minutes

Total Time: **10** Minutes

INGREDIENTS

- 2 grams cannabis
- 2 slices bread
- 2 slices cheese
- 2 eggs
- 2 slices bacon

DIRECTIONS

1. Cook the bacon and scramble the eggs.
2. Butter a slice of bread then add the ingredients however you like.
3. Microwave for 30 seconds.

GRILLED CHEESE SANDWICH

Serves: **4**

Prep Time: **10** Minutes

Cook Time: **10** Minutes

Total Time: **20** Minutes

INGREDIENTS

- 4 slices cheese
- 2 tbs cannabis-infused butter
- 4 tbs jam
- 1 pear
- Salt
- 4 slices bread

DIRECTIONS

1. Preheat a skillet.
2. Slice the pear.
3. Smear the bread slices with the cannabis butter.
4. Smear the other side with the jam.
5. Place the slice of bread, butter side down onto the skillet.
6. Place the pear slices and cheese on top.

7. Reduce the heat and cook covered for a few minutes.
8. Smear another slice of bread with the remaining cannabis butter and place it on top.
9. Flip over to cook on the other side for 3 more minutes.
10. Serve immediately.

HAM & CHEDDAR PANINI

Serves: 2

Prep Time: 10 Minutes

Cook Time: 5 Minutes

Total Time: 15 Minutes

INGREDIENTS

- ½ cup sauerkraut
- ½ cup peppers
- Arugula
- 1 tomato
- 4 ounces cheddar
- 2 ounces ham
- 2 pieces of baguette
- 3 tbs cannabis-infused oil

DIRECTIONS

1. Preheat a skillet.
2. Saute the peppers in the cannabis oil.
3. Layer the sandwiches with arugula, ham and tomato.
4. Top with cheese, peppers and sauerkraut.
5. Grill until the cheese is melted, serve warm.

WAFFLES

Serves: **4**

Prep Time: **10** Minutes

Cook Time: **10** Minutes

Total Time: **20** Minutes

INGREDIENTS

- ¾ cup milk
- ½ lb bacon
- 2 eggs
- ½ gr BHO shatter
- 2 tbs coconut oil
- ½ cup grated cheese

- Pancake waffle mix

DIRECTIONS

1. Melt the coconut oil.
2. Add the BHO concentrate.
3. Remove from heat.
4. Fry the bacon, then chop.
5. Mix the eggs into the coconut oil bowl.
6. Whisk, add the milk, and whisk again.
7. Bake the waffles using the waffle iron.
8. Serve immediately.

BISCUITS

Serves: 4
Prep Time: 10 Minutes
Cook Time: 15 Minutes
Total Time: 25 Minutes

INGREDIENTS

- 1 tsp salt
- Black pepper

- 3 cloves garlic
- 2/3 cup coconut flour
- ½ cup cannabis-infused coconut oil
- 6 eggs
- 1 cup cheese
- 1 tsp baking powder

DIRECTIONS

1. Preheat the oven to 400F.
2. Sift the flour, baking powder, salt and pepper in a bowl.
3. Beat the oil and the eggs.
4. Add the garlic and cheese.
5. Combine the ingredients.
6. Drop by spoonfuls on a baking sheet.
7. Bake for 15 minutes.

CRISPY BACON

Serves: **4**

Prep Time: **10** Minutes

Cook Time: **10** Minutes

Total Time: **20** Minutes

INGREDIENTS

- 12 strips bacon
- 1 cup cantaloupe
- toothpicks
- 1 tbs shake flour
-

DIRECTIONS

1. Preheat the oven to 200F.
2. Place the bacon on the cookie sheet.
3. Cook until crisp.
4. Flip over and toss with shake flour.
5. Return to oven and cook until desired crispiness.
6. Wrap the bacon around the cantaloupe.
7. Refrigerate and serve.

MUNCHIE BALLS

Serves: **4**

Prep Time: **10** Minutes

Cook Time: **10** Minutes

Total Time: **20** Minutes

INGREDIENTS

- 2 tbs cocoa powder
- ¼ cup peanut butter
- 1 ½ cups cannabis-infused butter
- 3 cups rolled oats
- 3 tbs honey

DIRECTIONS

1. **Melt the cannabis butter.**
2. **Add the rest of the ingredients and cook for 5 minutes.**
3. **Spread the mixture into baking pan and refrigerate for 15 minutes.**
4. **Form balls and refrigerate.**

QUESADILLA

Serves: **4**

Prep Time: **5** Minutes

Cook Time: **10** Minutes

Total Time: **15** Minutes

INGREDIENTS

- 4 tbs cannabis-infused oil
- 4 ounces ham
- 8 slices dill pickle
- 8 tortillas
- 3 tbs mustard
- 4 ounces roast pork
- 4 ounces Swiss cheese

DIRECTIONS

1. Brush one side of the tortillas with mustard and the other side with the cannabis oil.
2. Divide the ham, pickles, pork and cheese on the tortillas.
3. Top with the remaining tortillas.
4. Grate for 3 minutes.

FOIE GRAS PATE

Serves: *8*
Prep Time: *10* Minutes
Cook Time: *3* Hours
Total Time: *40* Minutes

INGREDIENTS

- 1 quart glycerin
- 2 tbs glycerin tincture
- 1 lb gras lobe
- ½ cup Sauternes
- 1 ounce cannabis
- 1 cup heavy cream
- 1 ½ tbs salt
- ½ cup garlic
- ½ cup shallot confit
- 5 sheets bloom gelatin

DIRECTIONS

1. Preheat the oven to 230F.
2. Bake the cannabis for 30 minutes.
3. Preheat a slow cooker and add the glycerin.

4. Add the plant material and stir.
5. Cook covered for 3 hours.
6. Strain to remove the plant material.
7. Mix all ingredients in a blender.
8. Blend until smooth.

STEAK WITH CHIMICHURRI SAUCE

Serves: **20**

Prep Time: **10** Hours

Cook Time: **5** Hours

Total Time: **15** Hours

INGREDIENTS

- ½ cup garlic
- 2 tsp chili flakes
- 1 ½ tbs vinegar
- 2 tsp salt
- 7 cups oil
- 5 lb steak
- 10 cannabis leaves
- 3 tsp oregano

DIRECTIONS
1. Mix the chopped cannabis, garlic, oregano, salt, 4 cups oil, chili flakes, and vinegar for the chimichurri sauce.
2. Season the steak with salt and pepper.
3. Refrigerate overnight.
4. Heat the rest of the oil in a skillet.
5. Cook the steak to desired doneness.
6. Serve topped with the chimichurri sauce.

MUSHROOM BRUSCHETTA

Serves: 6
Prep Time: 5 Minutes
Cook Time: 15 Minutes
Total Time: 20 Minutes

INGREDIENTS
- 2 tsp salt
- 1 ½ tsp pepper
- 1 clove garlic
- 2 ½ tbs vinegar
- 3 cups mushroom
- A loaf of bread

- 4 tbs oil
- 1 tbs thyme
- 4 tsp cannabis-infused oil

DIRECTIONS

1. Heat the regular oil in a frying pan.
2. Saute the mushrooms for 2 minutes.
3. Add the vinegar and stir for 30 seconds.
4. Add the thyme, salt and pepper to taste.
5. Toast the bread and rub each piece with garlic, then drizzle the infused oil over.
6. Serve topped with the mushroom mixture.

GNOCCHI IN GANJA BUTTER

Serves: 4
Prep Time: 20 Minutes
Cook Time: 40 Minutes
Total Time: 60 Minutes

INGREDIENTS

- 3 cups flour

- 2 tsp salt
- ½ cup cheese
- 1 egg
- 3 potatoes
- 2 tbs oil
- 4 tbs cannabis-infused butter
- 1 ½ tsp baking powder

DIRECTIONS

1. Boil the potatoes in salted water.
2. Remove the skins and mash.
3. Mix all of the ingredients together.
4. Kneed the potato on a floured table until it resembles bread dough.
5. Cut the dough into sizes of a small thumb.
6. Cook them for 5 minutes.
7. Boil until they rise to the top of the water, then cook for another 5 minutes.
8. Remove from water and add the melted butter.
9. Serve warm.

CHICKEN PASTA

Serves: 2
Prep Time: 30 Minutes
Cook Time: *2h 30* Minutes
Total Time: 3 Hours

INGREDIENTS

- 1 egg
- ½ cup sugar
- 1 ½ cup breadcrumbs
- 3 tbs cannabis-infused oil
- 2 chicken breasts
- 1 cup marinara sauce
- 5 cups water
- 1 cup flour
- ½ cup salt
- 1 lb pasta
- 2 cups cheese

DIRECTIONS

1. Mix the salt and sugar in water.
2. Add the chicken and refrigerate for 3 hours.

3. Preheat the oven to 350F.
4. Dip the chicken in flour, stirred egg, then in breadcrumbs.
5. Heat the oil in a frying pan.
6. Cook the chicken until golden on both sides.
7. Spread the marinara sauce at the bottom of a pan.
8. Place the chicken on top, then cover with cheese.
9. Bake for 30 minutes, covered with aluminum foil.
10. Cook the pasta.
11. Serve the pasta topped with the chicken.

LOBSTER ETOUFFEE

Serves: 8
Prep Time: **10** Minutes

Cook Time: **50** Minutes

Total Time: **60** Minutes

INGREDIENTS

- 2 cup onion
- 1 15-ounces can tomatoes
- 2 tsp salt 5 lobster tails

- 1 cup green onions
- 1 cup parsley
- ½ cup oil
- 2 tbs cannabis-infused butter
- ½ cup bell pepper
- 4 garlic cloves
- 3 bay leaves
- 2 tsp pepper
- 4 dashes hot sauce
- 5 cups lobster stock
- ½ cup flour

DIRECTIONS

1. Melt the butter in a saucepan.
2. Whisk the flour into the oil and cook for 20 minutes until the mixture turns a caramel color.
3. Add the garlic, onion and bell pepper and cook for 5 minutes.
4. Add the pepper, green onions, hot sauce and parsley.
5. Add the lobster stock and tomatoes and season with salt.
6. Bring to a boil, then simmer for 15 minutes.
7. Add the lobster and cook for 5 minutes.
8. Serve garnished with green onions and parsley.

SHRIMP SCAMPI

Serves: 6

Prep Time: 30 Minutes

Cook Time: 10 Minutes

Total Time: 40 Minutes

INGREDIENTS

- 2 garlic cloves
- 2 tsp black pepper
- 2 lbs shrimp
- ½ lb Cannabis-infused butter
- 1 lemon
- 1 cup shallots
- 2 cups white wine
- ½ cup parsley

DIRECTIONS

1. Heat 2 tablespoons of oil in a pan and cook the shrimp.
2. Peel the shells off.
3. Add the butter to the pan and cook the shallots for 3 minutes.

4. Add the garlic and cook for another minute.
5. Add the white wine.
6. Swirl the remaining butter and add the shrimp.
7. Season with salt and lemon juice, serve warm.

STRIP STEAK

Serves: **6**
Prep Time: **10** Minutes
Cook Time: **10** Minutes
Total Time: **20** Minutes

INGREDIENTS

- 4 prime strips
- 1 cup cannabis-infused butter

DIRECTIONS

1. Season the steaks with oil, salt and pepper.
2. Preheat the grill.
3. Grill steaks for 3 minutes.
4. Allow to rest.

5. Serve with a scoop of cannabis butter.

HOT WINGS

Serves: **6**

Prep Time: **20** Minutes

Cook Time: **20** Minutes

Total Time: **40** Minutes

INGREDIENTS

- Ranch
- Cooking oil
- Hot sauce
- 2 lb chicken wings
- ½ cup cannabis-infused butter

DIRECTIONS

1. Heat the oil in a frying pan.
2. Add the chicken when the oil is hot enough.
3. Fry for 15 minutes.
4. Melt the cannabis butter in the microwave.

5. Mix the hot sauce with the butter.
6. Say ½ cup hot sauce and ½ cup cannabis butter.
7. Place the chicken wings in a bowl and pour over the cannabis hot sauce.
8. Serve with ranch dip.

MAC AND CHEESE

Serves: 2
Prep Time: 10 Minutes
Cook Time: 45 Minutes
Total Time: 55 Minutes

INGREDIENTS

- 4 cups milk
- 1 lb macaroni
- 2 ½ tsp salt
- 1 ½ tsp black pepper
- 1 cup flour
- ½ cup cannabis-infused butter
- ¾ cup breadcrumbs
- ½ cup butter
- 1 tsp cayenne pepper

- 4 cups cheese

DIRECTIONS

1. Melt the butter in a pan.
2. Add the flour gradually, whisking.
3. Add the milk in small batches, whisking.
4. Add the seasonings.
5. Take off the heat and add the cheese.
6. Add the cooked pasta and mix well.
7. Bake at 350F for 40 minutes.
8. Serve immediately.

TACOS

Serves: 6
Prep Time: **10** Minutes
Cook Time: **10** Minutes
Total Time: **20** Minutes

INGREDIENTS

- Taco shell

- Cheese
- Beans
- Onion
- Taco seasoning
- Salsa
- Cilantro
- Cannabis-infused butter
- Tomato

DIRECTIONS

1. Spread the cannabis butter over each taco shell.
2. Add taco meat and the cheese.
3. Bake at 350F until the cheese melts.
4. Add the desired toppings, serve hot.

BURGERS

Serves: 4
Prep Time: 20 Minutes
Cook Time: 10 Minutes
Total Time: 30 Minutes

INGREDIENTS

- 1 gram weed
- Salt
- 1 lb ground beef
- Pepper

DIRECTIONS

1. Mix the ground beef with the weed powder.
2. Shape the meat into patties.
3. Season with salt and pepper.
4. Grill for 5 minutes per side, serve on a bun.

SALAD

Serves: 2
Prep Time: 15 Minutes
Cook Time: 0 Minutes
Total Time: 15 Minutes

INGREDIENTS

- Spring onions

- Tomatoes
- Salt
- Pepper
- Marijuana leaves
- Mushrooms
- Cucumber
- 1 clove garlic
- Olives
- Basil leaves
- Oil
- Lemon juice
- Vinegar
- Lettuce

DIRECTIONS

1. Chop the marijuana and basil leaves.
2. Cut the vegetables and add to a bowl next to the leaves.
3. Peel the garlic and crush it down.
4. Chop it and put it in a bowl.
5. Add some chopped olives.
6. Add oil, lemon juice and vinegar.
7. Season with salt and pepper.
8. Mix well.
9. Pour the dressing over the salad.
10. Serve immediately.

TURKEY BOLOGNESE

Serves: **8**

Prep Time: **15** Minutes

Cook Time: **40** Minutes

Total Time: **55** Minutes

INGREDIENTS

- 1 can tomato sauce
- 1 ½ tsp pepper
- 10 drops cannabis tincture
- 3 carrots
- 1 onion
- 2 celery stalks
- 3 cloves garlic
- 1 box spaghetti
- 3 tbs oil
- 1 lb ground turkey
- ½ cup parsley
- 1 cup cheese
- 2 tsp salt
- 1 can tomatoes

DIRECTIONS

1. Heat the oil and cook the onion, celery and carrots until soft.
2. Add the garlic and turkey.
3. When the turkey is browned, add the tomatoes and tomato sauce.
4. Let simmer covered for 30 minutes.
5. Bring a pot of water to a rolling boil.
6. Add salt, then add the pasta and cook.
7. Toss the drained pasta in the cannabis tincture.
8. Add the Bolognese sauce on top and mix.
9. Serve topped with parsley and parmesan.

BATTERED FISH

Serves: 4
Prep Time: 20 Minutes
Cook Time: 30 Minutes
Total Time: 50 Minutes

INGREDIENTS

- 6 cups oil

- 1 tsp salt
- 3 tbs cane sugar
- 12 ounces beer
- 2 tsp baking powder
- 3 tbs cannabis-infused oil
- Hot sauce
- 1 lemon
- 1 ½ lb fish fillets
- 3 cups flour
- 1/3 cup cornmeal
- 3 tbs butter
- 1 tsp vanilla

DIRECTIONS

1. Whisk 2 ½ cups of flour, cornmeal, baking powder and salt.
2. Mix ¾ cup of the mixture with the remaining flour.
3. Whisk the sugar into the first flour mixture.
4. Mix 2/3 cup water with the melted butter and vanilla.
5. Add the wet ingredients into the flour-sugar mixture, and stir to combine.
6. Knead the dough on a floured surface for about 2 minutes.
7. Allow to rest for 10 minutes covered.
8. Divide the dough into 12 pieces and roll into ropes.
9. Heat the oil in a pot.
10. Fry the pieces of festival until golden.

11. Whisk the beer into the reserved bowl of flour and cornmeal.
12. Dredge the fish in the flour, then drop into the batter.
13. Fry until brown for 10 minutes.
14. Stir the cannabis-infused oil into the hot sauce to serve.

TUNA POKE BOWL

Serves: 4
Prep Time: 10 Minutes
Cook Time: 20 Minutes
Total Time: 30 Minutes

INGREDIENTS

- Diced tuna
- 1 avocado
- ½ cucumber
- 1 tbs ginger
- 2 tbs sriracha sauce
- 2 tbs seaweed
- 2 tbs sesame seeds
- 2 tbs lime juice

- 4 servings cannabis-infused oil
- 2 scallions
- 2 cups sushi rice
- 2 cups water
- 1 ½ tbs oil
- 2 tbs soy sauce
- 2 tsp salt
- 1 tsp sugar
- 2 tbs mirin
- 3 tbs vinegar
- 1 jalapeno

DIRECTIONS

1. Cook the rice in salted water for 15 minutes.
2. Mix the tuna, cucumber, avocado and jalapeno in a bowl.
3. Refrigerate.
4. Mix the soy sauce, vinegar, sesame oil, lemon juice, salt, lime juice, sriracha, sugar, ginger, rice wine and cannabis-infused oil.
5. Toss the tuna mixture into the sauce and allow to sit for 15 minutes.
6. Serve the rice topped with the rice, garnished with sesame seeds.

STEAK SALAD

Serves: **4**

Prep Time: **10** Minutes

Cook Time: **15** Minutes

Total Time: **25** Minutes

INGREDIENTS

- 2 bunches cilantro
- 1 bunch parsley
- 1 tsp mustard
- 2 tsp salt
- 1 ½ tsp pepper
- 20-ounces steak
- 1 bunch arugula
- 1 bunch scallions
- ½ cup carrots
- 15 cherry tomatoes
- 3 tbs cannabis-infused oil
- 1 tbs oil
- 2 tbs vinegar
- 1 lemon juice
- 1 ½ tbs chili powder

DIRECTIONS

1. Rub the steak with lemon juice and chili powder.
2. Grill, then allow to sit.
3. Combine the parsley, scallions, carrots, cilantro, arugula and tomatoes in a bowl.
4. Mix the cannabis oil, oil, vinegar and mustard in a separate bowl, then season with salt and pepper.
5. Serve immediately.

BAKED BEANS

Serves: **12**

Prep Time: **20** Minutes

Cook Time: **10** Hours

Total Time: **10h 20** Minutes

INGREDIENTS

- 5 tbs cannabis-infused oil
- 3 tbs mustard
- 4 cans beans
- 1 jalapeno

- 1/3 cup sugar
- 1 onion
- 1 cup BBQ sauce
- 1 cup ketchup
- 1 cup cooked pork

DIRECTIONS

1. Mix all of the ingredients in a crockpot and turn on low.
2. Cook for 10 hours stirring every 45 minutes.
3. Serve hot.

STUFFED POTATOES

Serves: 4
Prep Time: 20 Minutes
Cook Time: 20 Minutes
Total Time: 40 Minutes

INGREDIENTS

- Sour cream
- 4 tsp salt

- 1 bunch scallion
- 1 cup cheese
- 3 tsp pepper
- 5 strips bacon
- 2 potatoes
- 3 tbs cannabis-infused butter

DIRECTIONS

1. Preheat the oven to 350F.
2. Cut the potatoes in half, horizontally.
3. Scoop the filling out, and mash with the cannabis butter, seasoning with salt and pepper.
4. Cook the bacon until crisp.
5. Cook the scallions in the same pan for 3 minutes.
6. Top the potatoes with the scallions and chopped bacon.
7. Sprinkle with cheese and bake until melted.
8. Serve with sour cream.

SHRIMP QUESADILLA

Serves: 2

Prep Time: 15 Minutes

Cook Time: 25 Minutes

Total Time: 40 Minutes

INGREDIENTS

- 4 tortillas
- 1 cup cheese
- ½ cup bell peppers
- 6 shrimp
- 3 tbs cannabis-infused oil
- 2 ½ tsp oregano
- 5 tbs scallions
- 3 tsp salt
- 3 tsp pepper

DIRECTIONS

1. Heat the cannabis butter.
2. Saute the peppers for 5 minutes.
3. Add the shrimp and cook for another 3 minutes.

4. Add the scallions for 3 minutes, then remove to a bowl.
5. Place the pan on the stove and heat.
6. Add a tortilla and spoon half of the filling on top.
7. Sprinkle half of the cheese on top and cover with another tortilla.
8. Cook for 5 minutes, then flip over.
9. Cook for another minute, serve with salsa.

LUNCH

SPINACH, ARTICHOKE & MUSHROOM FETTUCCINE

Serves: **6**

Prep Time: **15** Minutes

Cook Time: **25** Minutes

Total Time: **40** Minutes

INGREDIENTS

- 2 cups baby spinach
- 1 cup cheese
- 3 tbs cannabis-infused butter
- 12 ounces fettuccine
- 1 onion
- 3 cloves garlic
- 1 tbs basil
- 1 15-ounces can artichoke
- ½ thyme
- 2 tsp salt
- 1 ½ tsp pepper
- 8 ounces mushrooms

DIRECTIONS

1. Combine the fettuccine, mushrooms, red pepper flakes, onion, garlic, thyme, basil, artichoke and 4 ½ cups water in a stockpot.
2. Season with salt and pepper.
3. Bring to a boil, then reduce to a simmer uncovered for 15 minutes.
4. Stir in the parmesan, spinach and the cannabis butter.
5. Serve sprinkled with parmesan.

QUINOA KALE SALAD

Serves: **4**

Prep Time: **15** Minutes

Cook Time: **20** Minutes

Total Time: **35** Minutes

INGREDIENTS
For the salad:
- ½ cup quinoa
- 5 cups kale
- ¼ cup sunflower seeds
- ¼ cup raisins
- 1 cup water

- 2 tbs cannabis-infused oil
- 2 chicken breasts
- 1 ½ tsp pepper
- ¼ cup cheese
- 1 tsp garlic powder
- 2 tsp salt

For the vinaigrette:

- ½ cup cannabis-infused oil
- 1 tsp honey
- ¼ cup lemon juice
- 2 garlic cloves
- 1 tsp salt
- ½ tsp pepper
- 1 ½ tsp oregano

DIRECTIONS

1. Put the quinoa in 1 cup of water in a saucepan and bring it to a boil.
2. Reduce to low and simmer for 15 minutes.
3. Cook the chicken in the heated cannabis oil for 10 minutes seasoning it with salt and pepper.
4. Allow to cool.
5. Toss together the kale, cooked chicken, sunflower seeds, quinoa and raisins in a bowl.
6. Whisk together all of the vinaigrette ingredients in a bowl.
7. Pour over the salad.
8. Serve topped with the parmesan cheese.

LEMON CHICKEN

Serves: **4**

Prep Time: **10** Minutes

Cook Time: **30** Minutes

Total Time: **40** Minutes

INGREDIENTS

- 1 ½ tsp pepper
- Rosemary
- 3 tbs cannabis-infused butter
- 5 tbs lemon juice
- 1 tbs honey
- 4 chicken breasts
- 3 tsp garlic
- 2 tsp Italian seasoning
- ½ cup chicken broth
- 2 tsp salt

DIRECTIONS

1. **Preheat the oven to 400F.**

2. Grease a dish.
3. Melt the cannabis butter in a skillet.
4. Cook the chicken for 5 minutes on each side.
5. Whisk the chicken broth, garlic, lemon juice, Italian seasoning, honey, and salt and pepper.
6. Pour over the chicken.
7. Bake for 30 minutes.
8. Serve garnished with rosemary.

SWEET CORN SALAD

Serves: 6

Prep Time: **10** Minutes

Cook Time: 5 Minutes

Total Time: 15 Minutes

INGREDIENTS

- ½ tsp salt
- 3 tbs cannabis-infused butter
- 1 tsp chili powder
- 6 ears of corn
- 3 tbs lime juice

- 1 tbs cilantro
- ½ cup queso fresco

DIRECTIONS

1. Boil the corn for 5 minutes.
2. Allow to cool.
3. Cut the kernels off the cob.
4. Whisk the butter, chili powder, cilantro and lime juice in a bowl.
5. Pour the mixture over the corn and mix.
6. Add the queso fresco and stir.
7. Season with salt and pepper, serve cool.

ROASTED MUSHROOMS

Serves: 4
Prep Time: 10 Minutes
Cook Time: 30 Minutes
Total Time: 40 Minutes

INGREDIENTS

- 1 ½ tsp pepper

- 2 cloves garlic
- 1 tbs oil
- ½ cup cannabis-infused butter
- 1 tsp thyme
- 1 lb mushrooms
- 1 tbs lemon juice
- 2 tsp salt

DIRECTIONS

1. Toss the mushrooms in the oil and season with salt and pepper.
2. Place on a baking sheet.
3. Cook for 20 minutes at 400F.
4. Cook the cannabis butter until brown.
5. Remove from heat and add the garlic, thyme and lemon juice.
6. Toss the toasted mushrooms into the butter and season again.
7. Serve immediately.

HOT WINGS

Serves: **4**

Prep Time: **20** Minutes

Cook Time: **40** Minutes

Total Time: **60** Minutes

INGREDIENTS

- 1 tsp garlic powder
- 5 ounces tomato sauce
- ½ cup hot sauce
- 25 chicken wings
- ½ cup cannabis-infused butter
- 1 ½ tsp chili powder

DIRECTIONS

1. Preheat the oven to 400F.
2. Bake the wings 25 minutes.
3. Melt the cannabis butter and mix with the tomato sauce, hot sauce, garlic and chili powder.
4. Toss the wings into the mixture.
5. Reduce to 250F and bake for 20 minutes.
6. Allow to cool, then serve.

BACON AND CHEESE POTATOES

Serves: **4**

Prep Time: **30** Minutes

Cook Time: **12** Hours

Total Time: **12h 30** Minutes

INGREDIENTS

- 1 lb bacon
- 5 tbs cannabis-infused butter
- 1 ½ tsp salt
- 2 onions
- 5 potatoes
- ½ tsp black pepper
- 1 tsp chili powder
- ½ lb cheese

DIRECTIONS

1. Line a slow cooker with aluminum foil.
2. Heat 1 tbs of cannabis butter in a skillet.
3. Add the bacon and cook until crispy.

4. Set aside to cool, then dice it.
5. Slice the onions and potatoes.
6. Grate the cheese.
7. Add the ingredients to the lined slow cooker, the rest of the cannabis butter, and top with cheese.
8. Season with salt, pepper and chili powder.
9. Seal up the foil and place the lid on the crick pot.
10. Cook on low for 12 hours, serve with sour cream.

BROCCOLI QUICHE

Serves: 6
Prep Time: 15 Minutes
Cook Time: 30 Minutes
Total Time: 45 Minutes

INGREDIENTS

- 2 cups cannabis-infused milk
- Salt
- Pepper
- 2 cups broccoli
- 2 tbs cannabis-infused butter
- 1 pie crust

- 2 cups cheese
- 4 eggs
- 1 onion
- 1 garlic clove

DIRECTIONS

1. Preheat the oven to 350F.
2. Melt the cannabis butter in a saucepan.
3. Add the garlic, onions, and broccoli and cook until soft.
4. Spoon the vegetables into the pie crust.
5. Sprinkle with the shredded cheese.
6. Pour the beaten eggs over and bake for 30 minutes.

SPINACH QUICHE

Serves: 8

Prep Time: 10 Minutes

Cook Time: 30 Minutes

Total Time: 40 Minutes

INGREDIENTS

- Pepper
- 1 onion
- 10 ounces spinach
- 3 cloves garlic
- 1 pie crust
- Salt
- 5 ounces can of mushrooms
- 6 ounces feta
- ½ cup cannabis-infused butter
- 8 ounces cheese
- 4 eggs
- 1 cup milk

DIRECTIONS

1. Preheat the oven to 375F.
2. Melt ½ cup of the cannabis butter.
3. Mince the garlic and chop the onion.
4. Add them to the skillet with the melted butter.
5. Cook for 5 minutes.
6. Drain the mushrooms and the spinach.
7. Chop the mushrooms and add them and the spinach to the skillet.
8. Add the feta and ½ cup of the cheese.
9. Season with salt and pepper.
10. Spoon the mixture into the pie crust.
11. Beat the eggs and the milk and pour the mixture over.

12. Bake for 15 minutes, then top with the remaining cheese and cook for 40 more minutes.
13. Allow to cool, then serve.

BUTTERNUT SQUASH SOUP

Serves: 4
Prep Time: 15 Minutes
Cook Time: 30 Minutes
Total Time: 45 Minutes

INGREDIENTS

- 3 lb butternut squash
- 1 tbs butter
- 1 tsp oil
- 5 cups chicken stock
- Nutmeg
- Salt
- Pepper
- 1 onion
- 1 red bell pepper
- 2 tbs cannabis-infused butter

DIRECTIONS

1. Cut the squash into chunks.
2. Melt the butter and oil in a pot.
3. Add the onion, red pepper and salt.
4. Cook for 8 minutes.
5. Add the squash and stock to the pot.
6. Bring to a simmer for 15 minutes.
7. Remove the squash and place in a blender, then pulse until pureed.
8. Season with salt, pepper and nutmeg.
9. Add the cannabis butter and stir, serve warm.

PUMPKIN POTATO SOUP

Serves: **4**

Prep Time: **10** Minutes

Cook Time: **15** Minutes

Total Time: **25** Minutes

INGREDIENTS

- 3 celery stalks
- 1 onion

- 5 cloves garlic
- 2 cups pumpkin puree
- 1 tsp nutmeg
- Salt
- 4 potatoes
- 3 tbs cannabis-infused oil
- Pepper
- 1 cup coconut milk
- 4 cups vegetable broth
- 2 tsp cinnamon
- 3 carrots

DIRECTIONS

1. Peel the potatoes, then cut them, the red onions and celery stalks.
2. Heat 2 tbs of cannabis oil.
3. Cook the potatoes and onions for 5 minutes.
4. Add the carrots and celery, stirring.
5. Cook for 5 minutes.
6. Add the minces garlic and season with salt and pepper.
7. Cook for another 3 minutes.
8. Add the remaining ingredients.
9. Bring to a boil, then simmer until potatoes are tender.
10. Blend until desired constancy.
11. Serve immediately.

TOMATO SOUP

Serves: **4**

Prep Time: **10** Minutes

Cook Time: **5** Minutes

Total Time: **15** Minutes

INGREDIENTS

- 1 tsp black pepper
- ½ red onion
- ½ lemon juice
- 3 tbs cannabis-infused oil
- 3 tbs vinegar
- 3 lb tomatoes
- 2 cloves garlic
- 2 tsp salt

DIRECTIONS

1. Combine the tomatoes with the garlic, lemon juice, salt and pepper.
2. Allow to sit.

3. Place the remaining ingredients in the blender and puree until smooth.
4. Allow to chill.
5. Serve topped with parsley and feta.

QUINOA STEW

Serves: **4**

Prep Time: **10** Minutes

Cook Time: **30** Minutes

Total Time: **40** Minutes

INGREDIENTS

- 1 cup bell peppers
- 1 cup zucchini
- 1 tbs lemon juice
- ½ cup scallions
- ½ cup quinoa
- ½ cup cannabis-infused oil
- 2 tsp coriander
- 1 tsp cumin
- 2 tsp oregano

- 1 tsp black pepper
- 3 cups vegetable stock
- 2 cups tomatoes
- 2 cups onion
- 2 tsp salt
- 1 cup potatoes

DIRECTIONS

1. Rinse the quinoa with cold water.
2. Heat the cannabis oil in a saucepan.
3. Add the onions, season with salt and cook for 5 minutes.
4. Add the drained quinoa, bell peppers, vegetable stock, coriander, oregano, potatoes, zucchini, pepper, cumin and tomatoes.
5. Bring to a boil covered.
6. Simmer for 20 minutes.
7. Stir in the lemon juice.
8. Serve topped with scallions.

CHILI CON

Serves: **4**

Prep Time: **30** Minutes

Cook Time: **2** Hours

Total Time: **2h 30** Minutes

INGREDIENTS

- 2 15-ounces cans black beans
- 5 tbs cannabis-infused butter
- 2 onions
- 10 plum tomatoes
- 2 15-ounces black-eyed peas
- 1/3 cup red wine
- 2 lb chopped beef
- 2 tbs cumin
- 2 15-ounces red kidney beans
- 2 ½ tbs chili powder
- 2 tbs chili flakes

DIRECTIONS

1. Place the beans in a pot of water under low heat.

2. When the steam begins to rise, add the wine and spices.
3. Add the tomatoes and onions after 45 minutes.
4. Fry the beef, adding the garlic into it.
5. Add the beef to the pot.
6. Cook the chili with weed for 2 hours, then blend the cannabis butter in, serve warm.

PEA SOUP

Serves: *8*
Prep Time: *30* Minutes
Cook Time: *2* Hours
Total Time: *2h 30* Minutes

INGREDIENTS

- 1 onion
- 2 garlic cloves
- 4 tbs miso paste
- 5 cups vegetable broth
- 5 cups water

- 4 cups split peas
- 4 tbs cannabis-infused coconut oil
- 1 ½ tsp thyme
- 2 carrots
- 1 ½ tbs cannabis-infused oil
- 2 bay leaves
- 1 ½ tsp salt
- 1 tsp black pepper

DIRECTIONS

1. Chop the carrots, dice up the onion and mince the garlic.
2. Place the carrots into a slow cooker.
3. Heat 1 tbs of cannabis oil, then add the onions and cook for 3 minutes.
4. Add the garlic and cook for 3 more minutes.
5. Add the onion and garlic to the carrots.
6. Add the peas to the slow cooker.
7. Season with salt, pepper, and thyme, then add the cannabis oil and miso paste.
8. Add the vegetable broth and water, along with the bay leaves.
9. Cook on high for 6 hours, stirring from time to time.
10. Serve topped with a sprig of thyme.

FRENCH ONION SOUP

Serves: **10**

Prep Time: **20** Minutes

Cook Time: **2h20** Minutes

Total Time: **2h 40** Minutes

INGREDIENTS

- 2 cups cheese
- 1 french baguette
- 4 tbs butter
- ½ cup red wine
- 6 onions
- 5 tbs cannabis-infused butter
- ½ cup water
- 8 cups beef broth
- 2 tsp salt
- 1 tsp black pepper

DIRECTIONS

1. Melt the cannabis butter and regular butter in a pot.
2. Slice the onions and add them to the pot.

3. Cook for 90 minutes, stirring often.
4. Toast the sliced baguette.
5. Pour the beef broth, water, red wine, salt and pepper into the pot.
6. Allow to simmer for 25 minutes.
7. Place the toast pieces in the base of 4 bowls.
8. Pour the soup in each bowl.
9. Top with shredded cheese.
10. Place the bowl into the broiler and cook for 10 minutes.
11. Serve garnished with thyme.

SPICY BURGERS

Serves: 4
Prep Time: 10 Minutes
Cook Time: 10 Minutes
Total Time: 20 Minutes

INGREDIENTS

- 4 slices cheese
- 2 gr bud

- 3 tsp oregano
- 4 hamburger buns
- 2 lb ground beef
- Salt
- Pepper
- 1 ½ tsp mustard
- 1 ½ tsp chili powder
- 2 tsp garlic
- 2 canned chipotle chiles
- 2 tsp salt
- 1 tsp black pepper

DIRECTIONS

1. Place all of the hamburger ingredients except for the cheese in a bowl.
2. Mix until well incorporated.
3. Divide into 4 patties.
4. Season the patties.
5. Grill for 5 minutes on each side.
6. Top the patties with the cheese slices during the last minute of cooking.
7. Serve on the buns topped with burger toppings.

VEGGIE TART

Serves: 8

Prep Time: 15 Minutes

Cook Time: 25 Minutes

Total Time: 40 Minutes

INGREDIENTS

- Salt
- 1 yellow pepper
- ½ cup cannabis-infused butter
- 1 leek
- 1 tsp cayenne pepper
- ½ bunch Swiss chard
- ½ cup cheese
- 1 tsp paprika
- 1 puff pastry sheet

DIRECTIONS

1. Preheat the oven to 450F.
2. Place the pastry sheet on baking sheet.
3. Heat the cannabis butter in a skillet.
4. Saute the leek and peppers for 6 minutes.

5. Add the Swiss chard and saute for 1 more minute.
6. Spread the vegetables across the pastry sheet and sprinkle the cheese on top.
7. Bake for 15 minutes, serve warm.

AVOCADO SHRIMP SALAD

Serves: 2

Prep Time: 5 Minutes

Cook Time: 5 Minutes

Total Time: 10 Minutes

INGREDIENTS

- 2 cloves garlic
- Pepper
- 1 avocado
- 10 shrimp
- 2 grapefruits
- 1 tsp honey
- 3 tbs cannabis-infused oil
- 1 red onion
- 1 lemon juice

- Salt

DIRECTIONS

1. Heat the cannabis oil.
2. Saute the garlic and onion for 5 minutes.
3. Add the shrimp and cook until pink.
4. Place in a bowl with the oil too, then add the remaining ingredients except for the avocado.
5. Toss, then top with avocado slices and serve.

GAZPACHO

Serves: 6
Prep Time: 20 Minutes
Cook Time: 40 Minutes
Total Time: 60 Minutes

INGREDIENTS

- ½ cup cannabis-infused oil
- 2 jalapeno peppers
- Salt

- Pepper
- 1 cucumber
- 5 tomatoes
- 1 red bell pepper
- 2 tsp garlic
- ¼ cup vinegar
- 5 ounces tomato juice

DIRECTIONS

1. Pulse the tomatoes, cucumber and bell pepper with a food processor.
2. Stir in the minced garlic.
3. In a bowl, mix the tomato juice, jalapenos, vinegar and cannabis oil.
4. Season with salt and pepper.
5. Mix everything together in the food processor.
6. Refrigerate before serving.

SNACKS, DRINKS & DIPS

MUDDY BUDDIES

Serves: **4**

Prep Time: **5** Minutes

Cook Time: **10** Minutes

Total Time: **15** Minutes

INGREDIENTS

- 1 tsp vanilla
- 1 ½ cup powdered sugar
- 9 cups Chex cereal
- ¼ cup butter
- 1 cup milk
- ½ cup cannabis-infused butter

DIRECTIONS

1. Mix the cannabis butter, butter and milk.
2. Remove from heat and stir in the vanilla.
3. Pour the cereal into a bowl and the chocolate sauce over.
4. Coat the cereal with the powdered sugar and spread on waxed paper to cool.

CARAMELS

Serves: **12**

Prep Time: **10** Minutes

Cook Time: **15** Minutes

Total Time: **40** Minutes

INGREDIENTS

- 1 tsp vanilla
- Salt
- 1 cup corn syrup
- 1 cup cannabis-infused butter
- 2 ¼ cup brown sugar
- 1 can condensed milk

DIRECTIONS

1. Melt the butter, add the brown sugar and salt.
2. Stir to combine.
3. Add the milk gradually.
4. Cook and stir for 15 minutes.
5. Remove from heat and stir in the vanilla.
6. Cool, cut and wrap.

FUDGE

Serves: **36**

Prep Time: **15** Minutes

Cook Time: **15** Minutes

Total Time: **30** Minutes

INGREDIENTS

- 1 tsp vanilla
- 1 cup cannabis-infused butter
- 1 ½ cups chocolate chips
- 4 cups sugar
- 1 ¼ cups milk
- 1 cup marshmallow creme

DIRECTIONS

1. Combine sugar, milk and cannabis butter in a pot.
2. Cook on medium for 12 minutes.
3. Remove from heat.
4. Stir in the chocolate chips, vanilla and marshmallow crème.
5. Stir until well mix.
6. Pour the mixture into the baking dish.

BROWNIES

Serves: **20**

Prep Time: **15** Minutes

Cook Time: **30** Minutes

Total Time: **45** Minutes

INGREDIENTS

- 1 cup cannabis-infused butter
- 2 cups chocolate chips
- 1 tbs vanilla
- 1 ½ cups cocoa powder
- 1 tsp salt
- 4 eggs
- 2 ¼ cups sugar
- 1 tsp baking powder
- 1 ½ cups flour

DIRECTIONS

1. Preheat the oven to 350F.
2. Mix the cannabis butter with the sugar in a bowl.
3. Add the eggs and vanilla extract
4. Beat until smooth.

5. Add the salt, baking powder, cocoa powder and flour to the egg mixture.
6. Stir in the chocolate chips.
7. Pour the batter into the pan and bake for 30 minutes.

COOKIE BARS

Serves: **4**

Prep Time: **10** Minutes

Cook Time: **30** Minutes

Total Time: **40** Minutes

INGREDIENTS

- 1 cup chocolate chips
- 1 cup graham cracker crumbs
- 1 can condensed milk
- 1 cup cannabis-infused butter
- 1 cup shredded coconut

DIRECTIONS

1. Preheat the oven to 350F.

2. Pour the melted cannabis butter into a baking dish.
3. Sprinkle the crumbs and press to form a crust.
4. Sprinkle coconut and chocolate chips over.
5. Pour the condensed milk over.
6. Bake for 30 minutes.

BROWNIE BARS

Serves: **16**

Prep Time: **10** Minutes

Cook Time: **30** Minutes

Total Time: **40** Minutes

INGREDIENTS

- 21-ounces brownie mix
- 2 eggs
- 2 tbs sugar
- 8-ounces cream cheese
- 1 tsp vanilla

DIRECTIONS

1. Preheat the oven to 350F.
2. Coat a baking dish with cooking spray.
3. Combine the eggs, sugar, and vanilla and beat with an electric beater.
4. Bake for 40 minutes, allow to cool then cut.

INDIAN BHANG

Serves: 2
Prep Time: 5 Minutes
Cook Time: 5 Minutes
Total Time: **10** Minutes

INGREDIENTS

- 2 tsp cinnamon
- 2 cups milk
- 3 grams butter
- 2 grams cannabis

DIRECTIONS

1. Melt the butter in a pan, add the cannabis and simmer for 1 minute.
2. Add milk, then add the cinnamon.

AVOCADO SHAKE

Serves: *1*

Prep Time: 5 Minutes

Cook Time: 0 Minutes

Total Time: 5 Minutes

INGREDIENTS

- ½ cup ice
- 3 tbs sugar
- 1 avocado
- 1 ½ cups cannabis-infused milk

DIRECTIONS

1. Blend all of the ingredients together.
2. Serve immediately.

BLUEBERRIES SMOOTHIE

Serves: **1**

Prep Time: **10** Minutes

Cook Time: **0** Minutes

Total Time: **10** Minutes

INGREDIENTS

- ½ tsp cannabis-infused honey
- 1 ½ cups chocolate milk
- ½ banana
- 2 dollops Greek yogurt
- 1 25-g packet Hemp Hearts
- 1 tbs peanut butter
- 1 handful blueberries

DIRECTIONS

1. Blend all of the ingredients together.
2. Serve cold.

HOT CHOCOLATE

Serves: **4**

Prep Time: **10** Minutes

Cook Time: **5** Minutes

Total Time: **15** Minutes

INGREDIENTS

- Cinnamon
- ½ gram cannabis
- 5 ounces chocolate
- 1 cup milk
- 1 cup light cream
- ½ tsp vanilla
- 5 tbs sugar
- Salt

DIRECTIONS

1. Mix the milk, sugar, and salt in a saucepan for 3-5 minutes.
2. Add the cream, vanilla, cinnamon and chopped cannabis.
3. Bring to almost a boil and add the chocolate.

4. Remove from heat and stir.
5. Serve topped with your favorite toppings.

ICED TEA

Serves: 6
Prep Time: 10 Minutes
Cook Time: 0 Minutes
Total Time: 10 Minutes

INGREDIENTS

- 5 tbs cannabis-infused butter
- 8 cups boiling water
- ½ cup sugar
- 6 chai tea bags
- 1 can condensed milk

DIRECTIONS

1. Place the tea bags in a pitcher.
2. Pour the boiling water over.
3. Remove the tea bags and add the sugar.
4. Allow to cool.

5. Mix the condensed milk with the melted butter.
6. Fill the glasses with ice cubes.
7. Fill the glasses with the tea and top with the condensed milk, stir and serve.

CARROT, BEET JUICE

Serves: 2
Prep Time: **10** Minutes
Cook Time: **0** Minutes
Total Time: **10** Minutes

INGREDIENTS

- ½ ginger
- 1 tbs cannabis-infused tincture
- 1 clove garlic
- 1 orange
- 5 carrots
- 1 beet
- 1 apple
- 1 lemon

DIRECTIONS

1. Chop the carrots, beets and apple.
2. Place the beet chunks into a juicer and process.
3. Add the garlic and ½ of fresh ginger.
4. Add the lemon and orange.
5. Pour the juice in a mason jar.
6. Add 1 tbs of the cannabis tincture and mix.
7. Serve immediately.

BLOODY MARY

Serves: *1*
Prep Time: *10* Minutes
Cook Time: *0* Minutes
Total Time: *10* Minutes

INGREDIENTS

- 1 tbs lime juice
- Ice
- 4 ounces tomato juice
- 2 ounces cannabis vodka
- 1 tbs Worcestershire sauce

DIRECTIONS

1. Shake together all of the ingredients.
2. Pour into a tall glass.
3. Serve garnished with olives.

COCONANABERRY SMOOTHIE

Serves: 2

Prep Time: 10 Minutes

Cook Time: 5 Minutes

Total Time: 15 Minutes

INGREDIENTS

- 2 cups milk
- 2 cups strawberries
- 2 tbs cannabis-infused oil
- 1 banana
- 4 tbs pomegranate juice

DIRECTIONS

1. Heat the cannabis oil in a skillet.
2. Saute the banana for 5 minutes.
3. Allow to cool.
4. Blend all of the ingredients, then add the banana.
5. Puree until smooth and serve.

MARTINI

Serves: 1
Prep Time: 5 Minutes
Cook Time: 0 Minutes
Total Time: 5 Minutes

INGREDIENTS

- 2 ounces cannabis-infused gin
- 1 cap dry vermouth
- ice

DIRECTIONS

1. mix the ingredients by stirring.

2. Serve garnished as you desire.

VANILLA MILKSHAKE

Serves: 2

Prep Time: *10* Minutes

Cook Time: *0* Minutes

Total Time: *10* Minutes

INGREDIENTS

- 2 tsp vanilla
- 1 ¾ cups cannabis-infused milk
- 4 cups vanilla ice cream
- 8 tbs sugar

DIRECTIONS

1. Blend all of the ingredients together.
2. Serve in a tall glass.

APPLE CIDER

Serves: 2

Prep Time: **10** Minutes

Cook Time: **5** Minutes

Total Time: **15** Minutes

INGREDIENTS

- 6 cups apple cider
- ¼ cup brown sugar
- 5 tbs lemon juice
- 5 cinnamon sticks
- 2 cups apple brandy
- Nutmeg
- 4 tbs cannabis-infused butter

DIRECTIONS

1. Add the cannabis butter, brown sugar and apple brandy in a pot and bring to a simmer until the sugar and butter have melted.
2. Stir in the cider, lemon juice and cinnamon sticks.
3. Bring to a boil.
4. Allow to cool, then serve garnished with nutmeg.

PEAR PROSECCO

Serves: **1**

Prep Time: **10** Minutes

Cook Time: **0** Minutes

Total Time: **10** Minutes

INGREDIENTS

- 10 mg cannabis tincture
- 2 parts prosecco
- 2 parts pear nectar
- 1 part cranberry juice

DIRECTIONS

1. Combine the pear nectar and cranberry juice.
2. Add the cannabis tincture and stir.
3. Pour the prosecco over.
4. Serve garnished with pear slices.

CANNABIS SYRUP

Serves: **4**

Prep Time: **10** Minutes

Cook Time: **10** Minutes

Total Time: **20** Minutes

INGREDIENTS

- 3 tbs chopped cannabis
- 3 cups sugar
- 3 cups water
- 2 tbs vegetable glycerin

DIRECTIONS

1. Mix the water and the sugar in a pot.
2. Boil until the sugar dissolves.
3. Add the glycerin and lower to a simmer, then add the cannabis.
4. Simmer for 5 minutes.
5. Strain and store

PEANUT BUTTER MILKSHAKE

Serves: 2
Prep Time: 10 Minutes
Cook Time: 0 Minutes
Total Time: 10 Minutes

INGREDIENTS

- Peanut butter syrup
- 1 ¾ cups cannabis milk
- 4 shots bourbon
- 4 cups peanut butter ice cream
- 4 tbs sugar
- Chocolate syrup

DIRECTIONS

1. Blend the ice cream, bourbon, sugar and milk together.
2. Spoon into glasses and top with syrups.

NUT BUTTER

Serves: **4**

Prep Time: **5** Minutes

Cook Time: **0** Minutes

Total Time: **5** Minutes

INGREDIENTS

- Nut butter
- Cannabis-infused oil

DIRECTIONS

1. Stir the cannabis oil into the nut butter.
2. Serve.

STRAWBERRY JAM

Serves: **2**

Prep Time: **10** Minutes

Cook Time: **25** Minutes

Total Time: **35** Minutes

INGREDIENTS

- ½ cup cannabis-infused honey
- ¼ cup lemon juice
- 3 cups sugar
- 4 cups strawberries

DIRECTIONS

1. Pour the honey into the glasses.
2. Cook the sugar and the lemon juice for 10 minutes.
3. Add the strawberries and cook for another 20 minutes.
4. Pour the mixture into the jars and mix with the honey.
5. Serve immediately.

VINAIGRETTE

Serves: 2

Prep Time: 10 Minutes

Cook Time: 0 Minutes

Total Time: 10 Minutes

INGREDIENTS

- 2 cloves garlic
- ¾ cup cannabis-infused oil
- ½ tsp oregano
- 2 tsp mustard
- Salt
- Pepper
- ¾ cup balsamic vinegar

DIRECTIONS

1. Blend all of the ingredients together.
2. Store in the refrigerator.

SALAD DRESSING

Serves: **12**

Prep Time: **10** Minutes

Cook Time: **0** Minutes

Total Time: **10** Minutes

INGREDIENTS

- 2 cups cannabis-infused oil
- 2 eggs
- ½ cup lemon juice
- 10 cloves garlic
- 3 tsp salt

DIRECTIONS

1. Place the eggs into boiling water for 30 seconds.
2. Crack the eggs into a blender.
3. Add the garlic, lemon juice and salt and blend, adding the cannabis oil.

GUACAMOLE

Serves: **4**

Prep Time: **10** Minutes

Cook Time: **0** Minutes

Total Time: **10** Minutes

INGREDIENTS

- 2 tomatoes
- 2 tsp salt
- ½ cup onion
- 2 tsp garlic
- 2 tsp cannabis-infused oil
- 3 avocados
- 1 lime
- Cayenne pepper
- 3 tbs cilantro
- 2 tsp cannabis

DIRECTIONS

1. Mash the avocado, lime juice, cannabis oil and salt.
2. Stir in the onions, cilantro, cannabis, tomatoes and garlic.

3. Add the cayenne pepper, refrigerate and serve.

CUCUMBER DIP

Serves: **8**

Prep Time: **10** Minutes

Cook Time: **0** Minutes

Total Time: **10** Minutes

INGREDIENTS

- ¼ cup cannabis-infused oil
- ¼ cup basil leaves
- 2 tbs dill
- 2 tbs tahini
- 2 cloves garlic
- 1 lemon juice
- 1 cucumber
- ¾ tsp salt
- 1 avocado
- ½ cup silken tofu

DIRECTIONS

1. Process the cucumber until smooth.
2. Add the rest of the ingredients and blend.
3. Season and serve.

CANNAQUESO DIP

Serves: 2
Prep Time: 10 Minutes
Cook Time: 15 Minutes
Total Time: 25 Minutes

INGREDIENTS

- 1 tbs salsa
- 1 ½ tbs butter
- 1 tbs cornstarch
- 8 gr cannabis
- ¾ cup sour cream
- 1 cup cheese

DIRECTIONS

1. Grind the cannabis.

2. Melt the butter, then add the cannabis and stir for 5 minutes.
3. Strain and return the butter to the pan.
4. Mix in the cornstarch.
5. Stir in the sour cream.
6. When hot and bubbly, add the cheese and salsa.
7. Stir for 10 more minutes.

HUMMUS

Serves: **8**

Prep Time: **5** Minutes

Cook Time: **5** Minutes

Total Time: **10** Minutes

INGREDIENTS

- 2 tbs water
- Salt
- Pepper
- 2 garlic cloves
- ½ cup cannabis-infused oil
- ½ cup tahini

- ¼ cup lemon juice
- 15 ounces can of chickpeas
- ½ cup cumin

DIRECTIONS

1. Blend the lemon juice and tahini for 40 seconds.
2. Add the garlic, chickpeas, cannabis oil, water and cumin.
3. Blend until smooth.
4. Store in the refrigerator.

SPINACH DIP

Serves: **4**

Prep Time: **10** Minutes

Cook Time: **4** Hours

Total Time: **4h 10** Minutes

INGREDIENTS

- ½ tsp salt
- 1 tsp pepper
- ½ cup cannabis-infused mayonnaise

- 1 cup cheese
- 10 ounces spinach
- 14 ounces can artichoke hearts
- ½ cup alfredo sauce

DIRECTIONS

1. Cook the ingredients in a slow cooker for 4 hours.
2. Serve with your favorite accompaniments

BLUE CHEESE DIP

Serves: 3

Prep Time: 10 Minutes

Cook Time: 0 Minutes

Total Time: 10 Minutes

INGREDIENTS

- ½ cup cannabis-infused butter
- 1 cup ranch dressing
- 1 cup blue cheese
- ½ cup sour cream
- 3 tbs milk

- 1 tbs hot pepper sauce
- ½ tsp cayenne

DIRECTIONS

1. Whisk all of the ingredients until well combined.
2. Serve immediately.

THANK YOU FOR READING THIS BOOK!

CPSIA information can be obtained
at www.ICGtesting.com
Printed in the USA
LVHW091914030620
657321LV00002B/261